No More Stretch Marks

The Most Effective and Simple Solutions to Get Rid of Stretch Marks

Elizabeth Grace

Table of Contents

Introduction

Chapter 1 - What can you Do About your Stretch Marks?

Chapter 2 - The Basics of Stretch Mark Removal

Chapter 3 - Find the Right Treatment for You: Natural and Non-invasive Solutions you can Prepare at Home

Chapter 4 - Alternative Stretch Mark Solutions (Invasive and Non-invasive)

Conclusion

Introduction

I want to thank you and congratulate you for purchasing the book, *"No More Stretch Marks: The Most Effective and Simple Solutions to Get Rid of Stretch Marks"*.

This book contains proven steps and strategies on how to treat your stretch marks, and how to prevent these stretch marks from forming.

This book will contain many natural and cost-effective remedies that can help you get rid of these unwanted marks. This book will also give you your much needed information about the currently available stretch mark treatment options. Now you can be more knowledgeable about how these stretch marks are formed. This book can even help you determine which stretch mark remedy is the best for you.

Thanks again for purchasing this book, I hope you enjoy it!

© Copyright 2015 by Elizabeth Grace - All rights reserved.

This document is geared towards providing exact and reliable information in regards to the topic and issue covered. The publication is sold with the idea that the publisher is not required to render accounting, officially permitted, or otherwise, qualified services. If advice is necessary, legal or professional, a practiced individual in the profession should be ordered.

- From a Declaration of Principles which was accepted and approved equally by a Committee of the American Bar Association and a Committee of Publishers and Associations.

In no way is it legal to reproduce, duplicate, or transmit any part of this document in either electronic means or in printed format. Recording of this publication is strictly prohibited and any storage of this document is not allowed unless with written permission from the publisher. All rights reserved.

The information provided herein is stated to be truthful and consistent, in that any liability, in terms of inattention or otherwise, by any usage or abuse of any policies, processes, or directions contained within is the solitary and utter responsibility of the recipient reader. Under no circumstances will any legal responsibility or blame be held against the publisher for any reparation, damages, or monetary loss due to the information herein, either directly or indirectly.

Respective authors own all copyrights not held by the publisher.

The information herein is offered for informational purposes solely, and is universal as so. The presentation of the information is without contract or any type of guarantee assurance.

The trademarks that are used are without any consent, and the publication of the trademark is without permission or backing by the trademark owner. All trademarks and brands within this book are for clarifying purposes only and are the owned by the owners themselves, not affiliated with this document.

Chapter 1 - What can you Do About your Stretch Marks?

Stretch marks can get quite unsightly if you do not treat them as soon as possible. Though this is a very common problem, especially with pregnant women and people losing weight, both men and women can benefit from various remedies that can improve the look of their stretch marks. Some of these solutions may even eliminate the whole problem if you manage to treat those marks fast enough.

Make sure to stay faithful to your chosen anti-stretch mark routine to yield the best results. You can find these solutions easily. Some of these solutions may even be available in your own kitchen, so you can get started immediately without having to spend a fortune.

Try to get to know your skin and how it reacts to various products. Some people are lucky enough to get great and fast results with simple and natural home remedies, some of which you can find in this eBook. Some people however may have deeper and older stretch marks that can take more time and money to treat. Some of these options are listed in this book. Keep in mind that some natural stretch mark remedies are potent enough to fade any kind of stretch marks, as long as you give them some time to do them work. Do not try to rush the healing process. Even laser treatments take time.

Stretch mark prevention is also important. If you find that your skin is prone to getting these marks, you may have to create a more intensive moisturizing routine. Target the spots where the stretch marks occur, and always keep some lotion or cream close by. Moisturizing is a great habit to have.

Stretch marks can be hard to remove, but with a little bit more patience, you may just see the results that you want. Eliminating these unsightly marks takes some time. Do not get discouraged if you do not see instant results. You will just have to keep on going until you see the improvement. By not ceasing your anti-stretch mark treatments, you can make your overall skin health much better; thus, preventing more stretch marks from forming in the future.

Keep your body stretch mark free with the help of "No More Stretch Marks: The Most Effective and Simple Solutions to Get Rid of Stretch Marks", so you can say hello to smoother and firmer skin in no time.

Chapter 2 - The Basics of Stretch Mark Removal

Tip Number 1: Moisturize regularly

Hydrated skin looks smoother and plumper, and they can help disguise the appearance of these pesky stretch marks. Remember to moisturize right after taking a bath. Some soaps and hot water can actually strip your skin of moisture, which can exacerbate the look of your stretch marks. Your favorite moisturizer will do.

If you think your stretch marks needs more hydration, you can choose a thicker cream. Massage the affected areas for at least a minute. You are not only hydrating your skin, but you are also gradually diminishing the amount of stretch marks that you can see on your skin by stimulating its natural collagen production.

Tip Number 2: Drink a lot of water

Skin needs to be hydrated to stay in perfect condition. Stay hydrated inside and out by drinking more than the recommended eight glasses of water. You will see great results, and your skin will look smoother and suppler. Drinking water will help you respond to these stretch mark treatments better, and you may even experience great results in a shorter period of time.

Your water intake will greatly influence the condition of your skin. Cut down on the unhealthy sugary drinks and go for those that really hydrate your body. You will see that you will have less skin problems to deal with if you drink more water or tea or fresh juices. Think of it as both a stretch mark treatment and prevention.

Tip Number 3: Exfoliate regularly

Scrubbing your skin regularly can help increase your cells' turnover rate, which means you will get fresher looking skin all the time. By exfoliating, you can gradually rid yourself of those deep jagged lines, or at least, make them look less prominent. If the stretch marks are not that deep, you can use scrubs that you can find in the drug store.

You may also use your loofah. Massage the affected areas, using a circular motion. This will give you smoother, stretch mark free skin after some time. The results will not be as fast as you think, but you really can improve your skin's texture if you keep to this routine faithfully. Remember that healing your skin will take some time, especially if you go for natural skin remedies.

Chapter 3 - Find the Right Treatment for You: Natural and Non-invasive Solutions you can Prepare at Home

Treatment Tip #1: Cocoa butter

Cocoa butter is a popular and inexpensive way to get rid of stretch marks, and it can also prevent any more of these unsightly marks from appearing if you apply it to your skin every day. This is such a great way to treat stretch marks since it is a natural fat substance that is compatible with the human skin.

Rub it onto the affected area once or twice a day, and preferably once before you go to bed. It will make your skin look plumper and you will also notice that your skin will feel much firmer in just one month of use. It also has that pleasant smell that most people are bound to appreciate.

Cocoa butter is easy to apply and makes less of a mess than oils, since it is solid at room temperature. You can easily melt the butter on your hands during application. You may also want to massage the affected area for a few seconds, although two to three minutes would be better.

Massaging the skin will help stimulate collagen growth, which can reduce the look of jagged stretch mark lines. You can get cocoa butter in organic shops, drug stores or online. You may want to go for pure organic cocoa butter for the best results.

Pregnant women may want to apply this to their skin even before they get stretch marks. Cocoa butter is great for stretch mark prevention. Remember that it is much harder to get rid of these stretch marks than preventing them from forming on your body.

Treatment Tip #2: Coconut oil

Coconut oil is usually considered as a miracle oil by many individuals, including beauty gurus. This oil has natural healing properties, and it can moisturize your skin like no other oil can. It lessens the harsh appearance of stretch marks by making the skin healthier and plumper.

Coconut oil can come in solid tub form as well as liquid form, and it is a very inexpensive all around treatment. You can apply this oil once or twice a day on the affected area. You do not have to put a lot of coconut oil on, and you do not need to be a greasy mess for this to work. A drop or two of this oil can give you great results already.

You can do this treatment for as long as you like, and you can even turn this into your regular moisturizer to prevent any recurrence of unsightly marks on your skin. It is definitely worth a try, since it is known as one of the best natural skin remedies and you can find this in grocery stores, drug stores and organic shops.

Treatment Tip #3: Vitamin E

Breaking up Vitamin E capsules and rubbing the liquid over scars and stretch marks is a common do it yourself procedure. It is also quite the popular choice for treating skin problems. You may do this once a day, every night, for as long as you want to do this treatment. You may also try doing this twice a day if you like. You can mix the Vitamin E liquid with your daily moisturizer to maximize its potential of getting absorbed by your skin.

Massage the affected area to stimulate collagen growth. You will see positive results in one to three months. To give yourself extra healing power, you may also like to take some Vitamin E as a supplement. You can take this once or twice a day. This is a cheap and effective do it yourself remedy, and you can find Vitamin E capsules just about anywhere. You may even have it in your medicine cabinet now.

Treatment Tip #4: Derma rollers

Derma rollers are fast getting a good reputation in skin care. This is a roller brush shaped apparatus covered with numerous micro needles. This works by stimulating the skin by micro-pricking. It encourages collagen production in your skin, thereby leaving it feeling plumper and fuller instantly. Many reviews show that you can experience great results within one month of regular use.

Using a derma roller may cause some minor bleeding. You will have to learn how to handle the rollers properly to reduce this, although the skin can easily adapt to this in time. You may also use serums or moisturizers to help the effects of the derma roller. The absorption of products in the skin is increased after derma rolling, so you may as well take advantage of this.

Try to go for natural products that contain no irritants. You must remember that derma rolling can irritate the skin during the first use. You may experience soreness and bleeding, but it is quite harmless. If you are fine with putting these micro-needles in your skin, then go for it. Just remember to disinfect your derma roller before and after use to prevent any infections from happening.

Derma rollers come in different needle lengths. It is easy to get intimidated by these, but you can look up reviews online to see if the shortest one with the .5 mm needles is enough for the kind of stretch mark that you have. Some stretch marks may require the longer 1.5 mm needles for visible results. It is recommended to roll at least once to thrice a week. Rolling excessively can damage the skin.

Once you start seeing the results, you can reduce the rolling to just once a week. That will be more than enough to maintain beautiful and smooth skin and prevent the formation of any more stretch marks in the future.

Treatment Tip # 5: Sunflower oil

Sunflower oil is a great stretch mark remedy. If your stretch marks are not too deep, then sunflower oil can help you reduce their appearance. The oil is not heavy on the skin, and repeated use of this oil will result to firmer and suppler skin. Since it is a lightweight oil, you can leave it on the skin like a moisturizer. You can apply this on your skin as often as you want, and for as long as you want.

Sunflower oil is also hypoallergenic, but if you want to be extra sure, you can perform a patch test before treating your stretch marks with it. Sunflower oil can be hard to find in some areas, so some people may not have this as an available option.

Treatment Tip #6: Olive oil

Olive oil is a nutrient rich oil that has been used for treating and moisturizing the skin for centuries. Olive oil can be easily absorbed by the skin, so take note that a little goes a long way. You do not have to get all greasy for this method to work. One or two drops of the oil will be enough for this treatment to work. Make sure to heat up the oil by massaging this into the skin. Two to three minutes of massaging this into the affected areas will give you great results, as this makes it easier for the skin to absorb.

Olive oil has great moisturizing and firming properties and it can diminish the harsh jagged edges of your stretch marks over time. It leaves your skin glowing after repeated use, too. Olive oil can also protect your skin from any more scarring and overstretching. Use this method for at least a month. If you like the results, you can use this for as long as you like. You can even use it on the rest of your body so make sure to remain stretch mark free.

Treatment Tip #7: Honey

Honey has great moisturizing and antibacterial properties that can help reduce the appearance of stretch marks. Honey is also a compound that can break down scar tissue, making it quite a potent stretch mark remedy. Most people reach for honey to make their skin looks firmer and smoother.

Make sure to use pure honey, and not the kind with added preservatives. Rub it onto the affected area once a day and leave it on for at least twenty minutes to an hour. You may also want to cover this up with some cling wrap to help get the honey absorbed into the skin faster. You will feel instant results. In a month, you will notice that your stretch marks look less prominent.

Treatment Tip #8: Honey and lemon

Honey and lemon are quite potent skin remedies. Lemon will help lighten the appearance of your stretch marks, visibly fading them within a month of use. Honey will improve your skin's texture, and it will help you to prevent any more stretch marks. You should apply this mixture to your stretch marks once a day. Leave it on for at least twenty minutes to an hour. Keep doing this treatment for a month or two.

Please remember that lemon can be slightly damaging to the skin, when used in excess, so you may benefit from giving your skin a break every now and then. Remember to moisturize after washing the mixture off.

Treatment Tip #9: Honey, salt and glycerin

This is another potent honey stretch mark treatment that you can do at home. You will have to leave this on for at least five minutes, twice a day for a whole month. To prepare this mixture, mix equal parts of honey, salt and glycerin. You can mix as much as you like, and if there are any leftovers, you can store it in the refrigerator for your next use. It will stay good for at least a week. You can easily rinse this treatment off with water. You may want to try this one in the bathroom if you do not want to risk leaving a mess and attracting ants inside your home.

Treatment Tip #10: Lemon

Lemon juice by itself is already a potent bleaching agent, which can fade the look of your stretch marks significantly in a short amount of time. You will also have to remember that plain lemon juice can cause the skin to dry up. You can try diluting this mixture in some water, and apply this to the affected areas with a cotton ball or a cotton pad. You can leave this on for a minimum of twenty minutes, or you can leave it on for an hour if you like.

Just take note that lemon can cause some stinging on the skin. Leave it on for as long as you can take it, and try not to force it to stay longer if it starts to hurt. You may end up burning your skin and leaving more unsightly marks. Remember to use sun protection on the affected areas during lemon treatment. Lemon can make the skin extra sensitive to UV rays.

Do this treatment three to four times a week for at least two months. It is important to give your skin a break every now and then, and always remember to moisturize after use. You can wash off the lemon juice on your skin with lukewarm water. Before applying this on your stretch marks, perform a patch test on your forearm so determine if you have any sensitivity to lemon juice.

Please remember to moisturize your skin after washing off the lemon juice.

Treatment Tip # 11: Coffee ground scrub with olive oil

Caffeine can help firm up the skin, while the grounds are exfoliating enough to soften jagged lines gradually and improve the overall look of the affected area. Mix this scrub with a bit of olive oil to double the results. You will get noticeably smoother and softer skin after your first use.

To make this scrub, take the used coffee grounds from your coffee maker, and mix it with a bit of olive oil. You can also put salt in this mixture if you like to increase your skin's healing abilities. Lessen the amount of olive oil if you want a rougher scrub. What is great about this do it yourself treatment is that you can customize it according to your own preference.

Massage this on to the affected areas for at least a minute. You can use this scrub for as long as you like, around three times a week to get great results. You will see that the lines will begin to soften in about a month's time and you get much firmer skin that is more resilient to stretch marks.

Treatment Tip #12: Aloe Vera

Aloe Vera is known for its ability to treat most skin problems. It is the best natural moisturizer, and the Aloe Vera gel gets readily absorbed into the skin. It is effective in minimizing scarring and it can also heal small tears in the skin. It is also cooling and soothing when applied, which is quite a nice sensation. It is not hard to find Aloe Vera gel. You can prepare your own Aloe Vera treatment straight from the plant, or you can buy some natural Aloe Vera gel in a bottle from your local drug store.

If you are taking the gel out of the plant, all you have to do it is cut a piece from the plant, split it open and rub the gel into your stretch marks. It is a simple process. You can leave the gel on for as long as you like, and you can rinse the gel off with lukewarm water afterwards.

Do not expect instant results with Aloe Vera. It may take months for you to see the results. Stretch mark removal is a long process, so you will have to persevere even if you are starting to feel like the treatment is not working.

Take note that Aloe Vera gel is not for everyone. Some people are allergic to it, so do a patch test before applying it all over your stretch marks. Just dab some gel on the inside of your arm and wait for an hour.

If you experience any signs of irritation or redness, it is best to find an alternative stretch mark solution. You may just be making another problem for yourself if you push it too hard.

Treatment Tip #13: Use a Stretch Mark Cream

There are so many stretch mark creams out in the market, but you can always check online, or ask your friends which one is the best one to get. If you check online, you will usually find dozens of reviews on a certain product. Look them up and weigh all of your options before committing to a product. It really is good to do your research beforehand so you minimize the risk of wasting money on a useless product. Like all the rest of these stretch mark solutions, it is best to apply these creams regularly, and try not to miss one day of it. Please remember to follow the instructions found on the label to get the intended results.

It will be good to review everything on the label before buying. You may find ingredients that can prove harmful to the skin. If a product contains harmful ingredients, then it is best to avoid using it. It is also important to do a patch test before smearing creams on your body. You may want to ask for testers so you can determine if you have any allergic reactions to a product before buying it.

Chapter 4 - Alternative Stretch Mark Solutions (Invasive and Non-invasive)

The stretch marks solutions listed in this chapter will need the guidance of a skin care professional. It would be best to avoid trying this by yourself to prevent any accidents.

Stretch Mark Solution #1: Laser Treatment

Going for laser treatments can be quite expensive, but they can get your skin to its pristine condition after just a few treatments. This kind of treatment applies heat to the skin to encourage the healing process. You must remember however, that one laser treatment will not be enough to make your stretch marks disappear. You will have to undergo a couple more sessions until they go away completely.

Most people go for less costly options for stretch mark removal, but if you have the cash, and if you want a sure way to get rid of your stretch mark problem, then this definitely is the way to go. It may be good to try creams and homemade solutions first, as you may get good results from these for much less.

Stretch Mark Solution #2: Use Retinoid Cream

You can go to a dermatologist to consult if retinoid creams are good for you and your skin type. These retinoid creams have shown dramatic results in treating stretch marks. It is quite potent, and it can be used for a couple of months. It is not recommended to start using this without the prescription of a doctor. You may get adverse side effects if you are not careful. This is not a natural skin remedy that you can put on without having to face consequences.

If you must try this cream immediately, you can perform a patch test on your forearm before applying this to other parts of your body. Try to determine if you have any allergic reactions to this kind of product before purchasing, as these creams can be very costly.

Stretch Mark Solution #3: Alpha Hydroxy Acid

The use of AHA, or alpha hydroxy acids produced some positive results on stretch mark removal. To be on the safe side, you may have to consult a doctor to check if this is compatible with your skin type. You may also like to patch test an AHA cream before going on with the full treatment, as some individuals can be allergic to this. Most AHA creams can come with rather high prices, so you may like to try before you buy.

Stretch Mark Solution #4: Glycolic Acid Peels

This is actually a great option for diminishing the appearance of your stretch marks. You can go to the dermatologist to have it done safely, but you also have the option to do it at home. Glycolic peels can be mild or strong. Stronger peels may require some downtime. Usually, with glycolic peels, you will need to do a few treatments before seeing the results. This might be worth the wait however, as glycolic peels can get into the skin deeper, making this a little more effective than most treatments. You will notice a change in texture and coloration within a month or two of regular treatments.

Take note that glycolic peels are not to be done all the time. You will have to rest for about a week or two before going for another treatment. Skin may become red and slightly irritated after treatment. It will be best to moisturize and wear sunscreen on affected areas. Wearing loose clothing near the treated parts may also help lessen the irritation.

Stretch Mark Solution #5: Microdermabrasion

Microdermasion is an effective treatment for white stretch marks. When stretch marks have fully matured and have settled into the skin, they usually become silvery or pale in color. Microdermabrasion can help improve the skin's texture by sloughing off the upper layer of the skin. The moderate exfoliation will also encourage the skin's collagen production.

If you think that this is the stretch mark solution for you, you should visit your dermatologist to get your first treatment. Microdermabrasion is a lot less costly than laser treatment or surgery, and it can yield great results after a few sessions.

Microdermabrasion treatment can be done once a month and you will see the results in less than a year. This is a safe and effective procedure as long as you get this done by a professional. Go to a clinic that you can trust.

Stretch Mark Solution #6: Skin Surgery

For severe stretch marks caused by drastic weight loss, your only option may be to go for skin surgery. Individuals may have to take time in considering this procedure. It is an invasive treatment that cuts out the scar tissue completely, making skin firmer and tighter. It also costs a lot of money.

If you only have the normal kind of stretch marks, it will be good for you to avoid having this procedure done. Recovery time is quite long, and you will have to wait for the surgery scar to heal completely.

Conclusion

Thank you again for purchasing this book!

I hope this book was able to help you to improve the look of your skin and your stretch marks.

The next step is to keep doing your chosen anti-stretch mark routine. It is best to be patient. You will see great results soon enough.

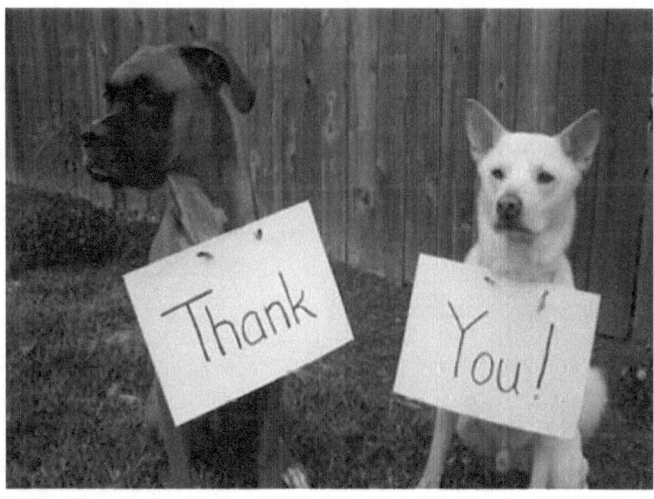

Finally, if you enjoyed this book, then I'd like to ask you for a favor, would you be kind enough to leave a review for this book on Amazon? It'd be greatly appreciated!

Thank you and good luck!